I0105931

This publication is intended to provide educational information for the reader on the covered subjects. It is not intended to take the place of personalized medical counseling, diagnosis, and treatment from a trained healthcare professional.

ISBN 978-1-998455-71-3 (Paperback)
ISBN 978-1-998455-72-0 (eBook)

Printed and bound in USA
Published by Loons Press

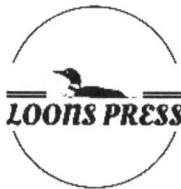

LOONS PRESS

Table Of Contents

Chapter 1	**6**
Understanding Cataracts	**6**
What are cataracts?	6
Causes of cataracts	8
Risk factors for developing cataracts	10
Chapter 2	**14**
Signs and Symptoms	**14**
Common symptoms of cataracts	14
When to see a doctor	15
Getting a cataract diagnosis	18
Chapter 3	**22**
Lifestyle Changes for Prevention	**22**
Importance of a healthy diet	22
The role of exercise in preventing cataracts	24
Protecting your eyes from UV rays	26

Chapter 4   **30**

Nutritional Strategies   **30**

Foods that promote eye health   30

Vitamins and supplements for cataract
prevention   32

Hydration and its impact on eye health   34

Chapter 5   **38**

Vision Care Practices   **38**

Regular eye exams   38

Proper eyewear for eye protection   40

Resting and relaxing your eyes   41

Chapter 6   **45**

Environmental Factors to Consider   **45**

Avoiding smoking and secondhand
smoke   45

Managing diabetes and other health
conditions   47

Limiting exposure to toxins and
pollutants   49

Chapter 7   **53**

Surgical Options for Cataracts   **53**

Understanding cataract surgery   53

Preparing for surgery   55

Recovery and post-operative care   57

Chapter 8   **61**

Support and Resources   **61**

Joining support groups for cataract patients   61

Finding financial assistance for cataract treatment   63

Additional resources for cataract prevention   66

Chapter 9   **70**

Conclusion   **70**

Recap of key strategies for preventing cataracts   70

Encouragement for maintaining healthy vision   72

Looking towards a future free from cataracts   75

Author Notes & Acknowledgments   **78**

Author Bio   **80**

How To Prevent Cataracts

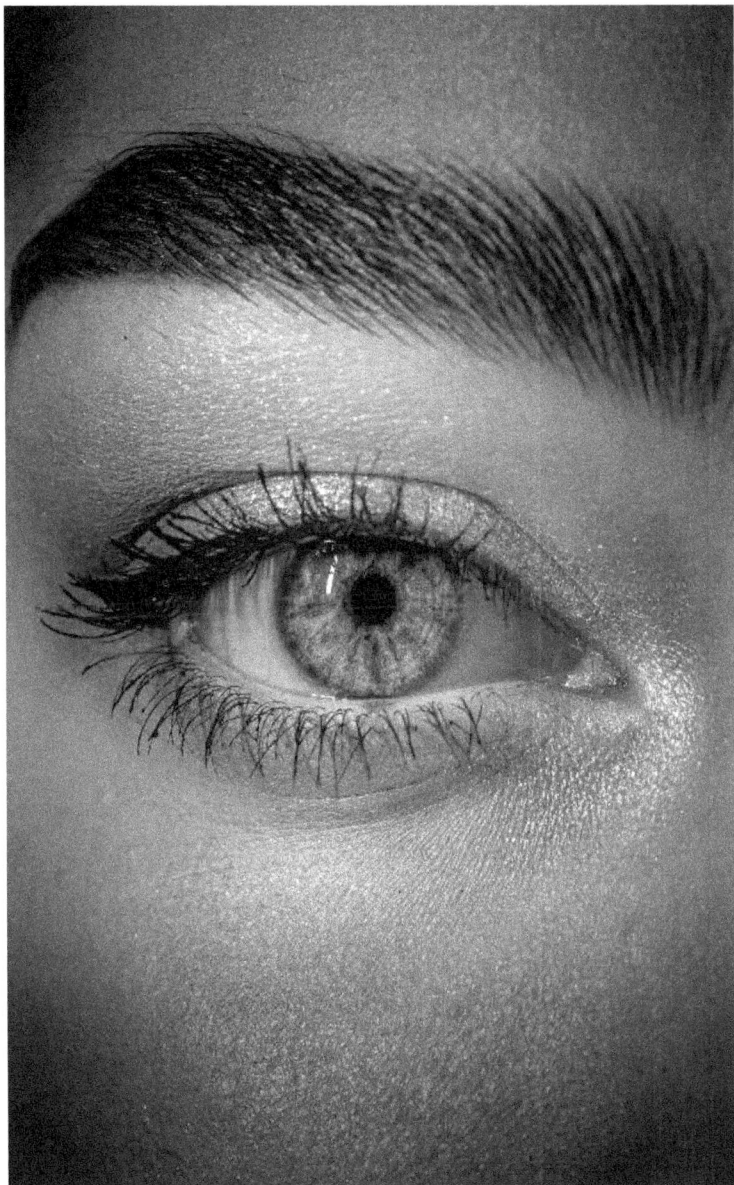

Chapter 1

Understanding Cataracts

What are cataracts?

Cataracts are a common eye condition that affects millions of people worldwide. They occur when the lens of the eye becomes cloudy, causing blurry vision and difficulty seeing clearly. Cataracts can develop slowly over time or can progress rapidly, depending on various factors such as age, genetics, and lifestyle choices. While cataracts are a common part of aging, there are steps that can be taken to prevent them from developing or worsening.

One of the main causes of cataracts is exposure to ultraviolet (UV) radiation from the sun. To prevent cataracts, it is essential to protect your eyes from UV rays by wearing sunglasses that block 100% of UVA and UVB rays. Additionally, eating a diet rich in antioxidants, such as fruits and vegetables, can help protect your eyes from cataract formation. Antioxidants help neutralize free radicals in the body, which can damage the eye's lens and lead to cataract development.

Another important factor in preventing cataracts is maintaining a healthy lifestyle. This includes not smoking, as smoking has been linked to an increased risk of cataracts. Regular exercise and maintaining a healthy weight can also help reduce your risk of developing cataracts.

It is also important to have regular eye exams with an optometrist or ophthalmologist to detect cataracts early and monitor their progression.

In some cases, cataracts may be caused by underlying health conditions such as diabetes or high blood pressure. Managing these conditions through proper medical treatment and lifestyle changes can help reduce your risk of developing cataracts. Additionally, certain medications, such as corticosteroids, can increase your risk of cataracts. If you are taking medications that may affect your eye health, speak with your healthcare provider about alternative options.

Overall, understanding what cataracts are and how they can be prevented is essential for maintaining clear vision and eye health. By taking proactive steps to protect your eyes from UV radiation, maintaining a healthy lifestyle, and managing underlying health conditions, you can reduce your risk of developing cataracts and enjoy clear vision for years to come. Remember, prevention is key when it comes to preserving your eye health and preventing cataracts.

Causes of cataracts

Cataracts are a common eye condition that affects millions of people around the world. Understanding the causes of cataracts is crucial in order to prevent or delay their onset. One of the main causes of cataracts is aging. As we get older, the proteins in our eye lens can start to clump together, leading to the clouding of the lens that characterizes cataracts. This process is natural and cannot be prevented, but there are steps you can take to reduce your risk of developing cataracts as you age.

Another major cause of cataracts is exposure to ultraviolet (UV) radiation. Prolonged exposure to UV rays from the sun can damage the proteins in the eye lens, increasing the risk of cataract formation. It is important to wear sunglasses that block 100% of UV rays whenever you are outside, especially during peak sun hours, to protect your eyes from UV damage.

Genetics also play a role in the development of cataracts. If you have a family history of cataracts, you may be at a higher risk of developing them yourself. While you cannot change your genetics, you can still take steps to reduce your risk of cataracts by maintaining a healthy lifestyle and protecting your eyes from harmful environmental factors.

Other factors that can increase your risk of cataracts include smoking, diabetes, and certain medications such as corticosteroids. Smoking can introduce harmful toxins into your body that can damage your eye lens, while diabetes can lead to high levels of sugar in the blood that can contribute to cataract formation. It is important to talk to your healthcare provider about any medications you are taking and how they may affect your eye health.

By understanding the causes of cataracts and taking steps to reduce your risk, you can help preserve your vision and maintain clear eyesight as you age. Making healthy lifestyle choices, protecting your eyes from UV radiation, and managing any underlying health conditions can all contribute to preventing cataracts and maintaining good eye health for years to come.

Risk factors for developing cataracts

Cataracts are a common vision problem that affects millions of people worldwide. While cataracts can develop for a variety of reasons, there are certain risk factors that can increase your chances of developing this condition. Understanding these risk factors is crucial in taking steps to prevent cataracts and maintain clear vision for as long as possible.

One of the primary risk factors for developing cataracts is age. As we get older, the proteins in the lens of our eye can start to break down and clump together, leading to the formation of cloudy areas known as cataracts.

How To Prevent Cataracts

While cataracts can develop at any age, they are most common in older adults, with the majority of cases occurring in people over the age of 60.

Another significant risk factor for cataracts is exposure to ultraviolet (UV) radiation from the sun. Prolonged exposure to UV rays can damage the proteins in the lens of the eye, increasing the risk of cataract formation. To reduce your risk, it's important to wear sunglasses that block 100% of UVA and UVB rays whenever you are outside, especially during peak sunlight hours.

Smoking is also a major risk factor for cataracts. The chemicals in cigarettes can accelerate the breakdown of proteins in the lens of the eye, increasing the likelihood of cataract formation. If you smoke, quitting can not only reduce your risk of developing cataracts but also improve your overall eye health.

Certain medical conditions, such as diabetes and high blood pressure, can also increase your risk of developing cataracts. These conditions can affect the health of the blood vessels in the eye, leading to changes in the lens and an increased risk of cataract formation.

Managing these conditions through proper medical care and lifestyle choices can help reduce your risk of developing cataracts.

In conclusion, understanding the risk factors for developing cataracts is essential in taking proactive steps to prevent this common vision problem. By addressing factors such as age, UV exposure, smoking, and underlying medical conditions, you can reduce your risk of developing cataracts and maintain clear vision for years to come. Taking care of your eye health through regular eye exams, a healthy diet, and lifestyle choices can go a long way in preventing cataracts and preserving your vision.

How To Prevent Cataracts

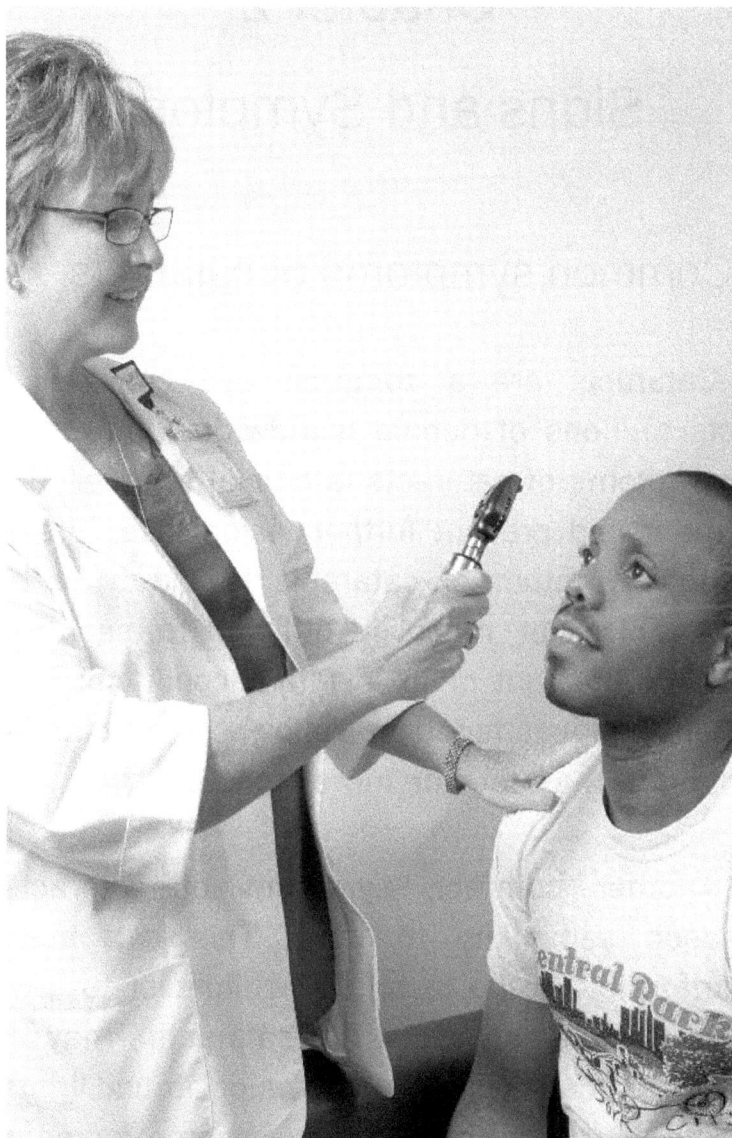

Chapter 2

Signs and Symptoms

Common symptoms of cataracts

Cataracts are a common eye condition that affects millions of people worldwide. Understanding the symptoms of cataracts is crucial in order to seek treatment and prevent further vision loss. The most common symptom of cataracts is cloudy or blurry vision. This can make it difficult to see clearly, especially at night or in low-light conditions. Colors may also appear faded or yellowed, and glare from bright lights may become more pronounced.

Another common symptom of cataracts is increased sensitivity to light. This can make it uncomfortable to be in bright sunlight or to drive at night. Some people with cataracts may also experience double vision or see halos around lights. As the cataract progresses, it may become increasingly difficult to read or perform other everyday tasks that require clear vision.

People with cataracts may also notice that their prescription for eyeglasses or contact lenses changes frequently. This is because the cataract causes the lens of the eye to become thicker and less flexible, affecting the eye's ability to focus properly. In some cases, cataracts can also cause a noticeable decrease in visual acuity, making it difficult to see objects clearly at a distance.

If you are experiencing any of these symptoms, it is important to see an eye care professional for a comprehensive eye exam. Early detection and treatment of cataracts can help preserve your vision and quality of life. In the next chapter, we will discuss strategies for preventing cataracts and maintaining clear vision as you age. Remember, taking care of your eyes is essential for overall health and well-being.

When to see a doctor

When it comes to eye health, it is crucial to know when to seek medical attention. If you are experiencing symptoms such as blurry vision, difficulty seeing at night, or seeing halos around lights, it may be time to see a doctor.

How To Prevent Cataracts

These can be signs of cataracts, a common eye condition that can lead to vision loss if left untreated. By seeking medical attention early on, you can prevent further damage to your eyes and potentially slow down the progression of cataracts.

If you have a family history of cataracts or other eye conditions, it is especially important to see a doctor for regular eye exams. Your eye doctor can monitor your eye health and detect any signs of cataracts early on. By catching cataracts in their early stages, you can explore treatment options and prevent further vision loss. Additionally, if you have diabetes or other health conditions that can increase your risk of developing cataracts, it is important to see a doctor regularly to monitor your eye health.

In some cases, cataracts can progress quickly and cause rapid vision loss. If you notice sudden changes in your vision, such as double vision or extreme sensitivity to light, it is important to see a doctor immediately. These can be signs of a more serious issue related to your cataracts, such as a detached retina or glaucoma.

By seeking medical attention promptly, you can prevent further damage to your eyes and potentially save your vision.

If you are considering cataract surgery or other treatment options for your cataracts, it is important to see a doctor to discuss your options. Your eye doctor can evaluate your eye health and recommend the best course of action for your specific needs.

By seeking medical advice, you can make informed decisions about your eye health and ensure the best possible outcome for your vision.

Overall, it is important to see a doctor if you have any concerns about your eye health or if you are experiencing symptoms of cataracts. By seeking medical attention early on, you can prevent further damage to your eyes and preserve your vision for years to come. Remember, your eye health is important, so don't hesitate to see a doctor if you have any concerns about your eyes.

Getting a cataract diagnosis

Getting a cataract diagnosis can be a daunting experience for many people who are concerned about their eye health. However, receiving a diagnosis is the first step towards effectively managing and treating cataracts. It is important to seek medical advice from an eye care professional if you suspect you may have cataracts, as early detection can help prevent further vision loss.

When visiting an eye care professional for a cataract diagnosis, they will perform a comprehensive eye exam to assess the health of your eyes. This may include tests such as visual acuity tests, tonometry to measure eye pressure, and a dilated eye exam to examine the lens for signs of cataracts.

The eye care professional will also take a detailed medical history to understand any risk factors you may have for developing cataracts.

After receiving a cataract diagnosis, the eye care professional will discuss treatment options with you. In the early stages of cataracts, simple lifestyle changes such as wearing sunglasses, eating a healthy diet rich in antioxidants, and quitting smoking may help slow the progression of cataracts.

However, if cataracts are significantly impacting your vision, surgery may be recommended to remove the cloudy lens and replace it with an artificial lens.

It is important to follow your eye care professional's recommendations for managing cataracts and attend regular follow-up appointments to monitor the progression of the condition. By staying informed and proactive about your eye health, you can take steps to prevent cataracts from worsening and maintain clear vision for years to come.

In conclusion, receiving a cataract diagnosis can be a scary and overwhelming experience, but it is an important first step towards effectively managing and treating the condition.

How To Prevent Cataracts

By seeking medical advice, undergoing a comprehensive eye exam, and following your eye care professional's recommendations, you can take control of your eye health and prevent cataracts from impacting your vision. Remember, early detection and treatment are key to maintaining clear vision and overall eye health.

How To Prevent Cataracts

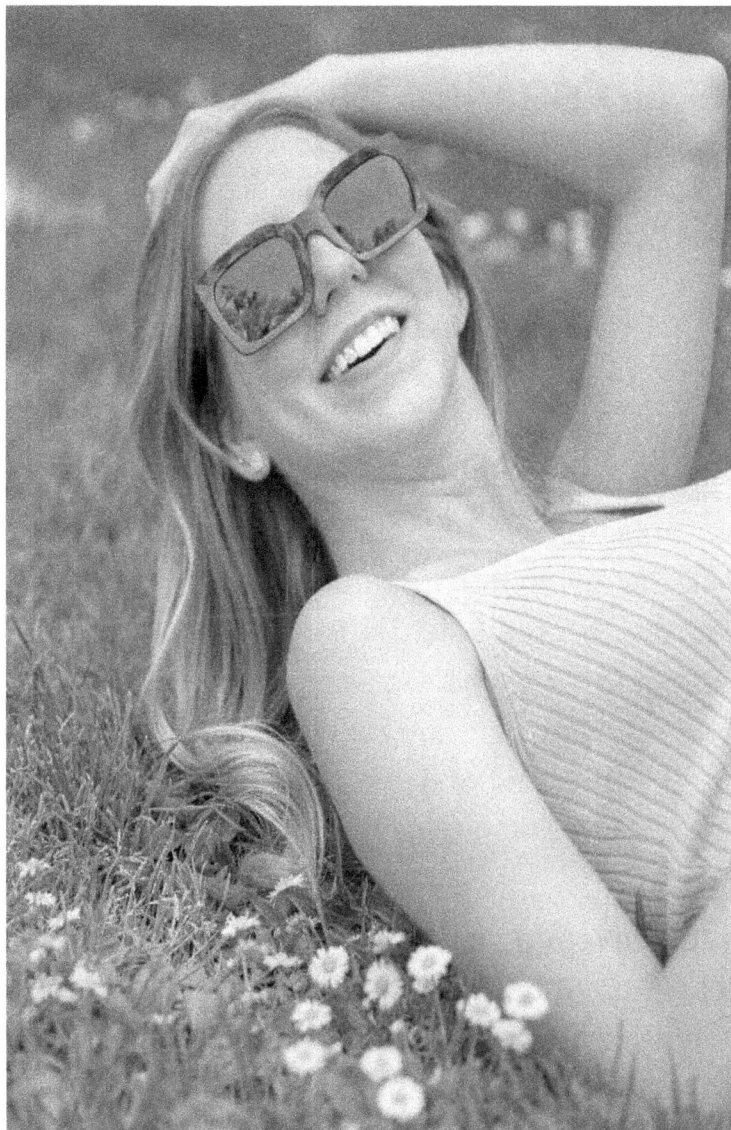

Chapter 3

Lifestyle Changes for Prevention

Importance of a healthy diet

Maintaining a healthy diet is essential for preventing cataracts and promoting clear vision. A diet rich in antioxidants, vitamins, and minerals can help protect the eyes from oxidative stress and damage caused by free radicals. By incorporating a variety of fruits, vegetables, whole grains, and lean proteins into your meals, you can support the health of your eyes and reduce your risk of developing cataracts.

One of the key components of a healthy diet for cataract prevention is consuming foods that are high in antioxidants. Antioxidants help neutralize free radicals in the body, which can contribute to the development of cataracts. Foods such as berries, leafy greens, and nuts are excellent sources of antioxidants and should be included in your daily diet to protect your eyes and maintain clear vision.

In addition to antioxidants, vitamins and minerals play a crucial role in maintaining eye health and preventing cataracts. Vitamin C, vitamin E, and beta-carotene are all important nutrients that can help protect the eyes from damage and reduce the risk of cataract formation. Foods like citrus fruits, almonds, and carrots are rich in these vitamins and can be beneficial additions to your diet for promoting clear vision.

A diet that is high in saturated fats, sugar, and processed foods can increase inflammation in the body and potentially contribute to the development of cataracts. By avoiding these unhealthy foods and focusing on whole, nutrient-dense options, you can support the health of your eyes and reduce your risk of cataracts. Incorporating foods like fish, olive oil, and whole grains into your meals can help reduce inflammation and promote clear vision.

Overall, the importance of a healthy diet for preventing cataracts cannot be overstated. By making smart food choices and prioritizing nutrient-rich options, you can support the health of your eyes and reduce your risk of developing cataracts.

Remember to include a variety of fruits, vegetables, whole grains, and lean proteins in your meals to protect your eyes and maintain clear vision for years to come.

The role of exercise in preventing cataracts

Cataracts are a common eye condition that can significantly impact one's vision as they age. While there are various factors that can contribute to the development of cataracts, such as genetics and age, engaging in regular exercise can play a crucial role in preventing their onset. Exercise not only helps maintain overall health and well-being but also has specific benefits for eye health that can help reduce the risk of developing cataracts.

Regular exercise has been shown to improve blood circulation throughout the body, including the eyes. This increased blood flow helps deliver essential nutrients and oxygen to the eyes, which can help prevent the formation of cataracts. Additionally, exercise can help lower inflammation in the body, which is a key factor in the development of many age-related conditions, including cataracts.

How To Prevent Cataracts

Incorporating a variety of exercises into your routine, such as cardiovascular exercises, strength training, and flexibility exercises, can have a positive impact on your eye health. Cardiovascular exercises, such as walking, jogging, or cycling, help improve circulation and lower inflammation.

Strength training exercises, like weightlifting or bodyweight exercises, can help maintain muscle mass and improve overall health. Flexibility exercises, such as yoga or stretching, can help reduce tension in the body and promote relaxation, which can benefit the eyes.

It is important to note that while exercise can be beneficial in preventing cataracts, it is just one piece of the puzzle. Maintaining a healthy diet, getting regular eye exams, and protecting your eyes from harmful UV rays are also essential steps in preventing cataracts.

By incorporating regular exercise into your routine and taking proactive steps to care for your overall eye health, you can reduce your risk of developing cataracts and maintain clear vision as you age.

In conclusion, exercise plays a critical role in preventing cataracts by improving blood circulation, reducing inflammation, and promoting overall health. By incorporating a variety of exercises into your routine and taking proactive steps to care for your eye health, you can significantly reduce your risk of developing cataracts. Remember to consult with your eye care provider before starting any new exercise routine, and make sure to prioritize your eye health as part of your overall wellness plan. With the right approach, you can maintain clear vision and enjoy a healthy, active lifestyle for years to come.

Protecting your eyes from UV rays

Protecting your eyes from UV rays is crucial in preventing cataracts, a common eye condition that can lead to cloudy vision and eventually require surgery to correct. UV rays from the sun can accelerate the formation of cataracts by damaging the proteins in the eye's lens. To protect your eyes from UV rays, it is important to wear sunglasses that block 100% of UVA and UVB rays whenever you are outdoors.

How To Prevent Cataracts

When choosing sunglasses for UV protection, look for a pair that has a label indicating they block 100% of UVA and UVB rays. Polarized lenses can also help reduce glare and improve visibility in bright sunlight. Additionally, wearing a wide-brimmed hat can provide extra protection for your eyes and the delicate skin around them from harmful UV rays.

It is not just sunny days that pose a risk for UV exposure - UV rays can penetrate clouds and cause damage to your eyes even on overcast days. It is important to wear sunglasses whenever you are outside, regardless of the weather. Remember to also protect your eyes from UV rays when participating in outdoor activities such as skiing, hiking, or water sports, as the reflection of UV rays off of snow, water, and sand can increase your exposure.

In addition to wearing sunglasses, it is important to eat a healthy diet rich in antioxidants to help protect your eyes from cataracts. Foods such as leafy green vegetables, fruits, nuts, and fish high in omega-3 fatty acids can help reduce oxidative stress in the eye and support overall eye health. Staying hydrated and getting regular eye exams can also help prevent cataracts and other eye conditions.

By taking steps to protect your eyes from UV rays, such as wearing sunglasses, eating a healthy diet, and getting regular eye exams, you can reduce your risk of developing cataracts and maintain clear vision for years to come. Remember, prevention is key when it comes to eye health, so be proactive in protecting your eyes from UV rays and other environmental factors that can contribute to cataract formation.

How To Prevent Cataracts

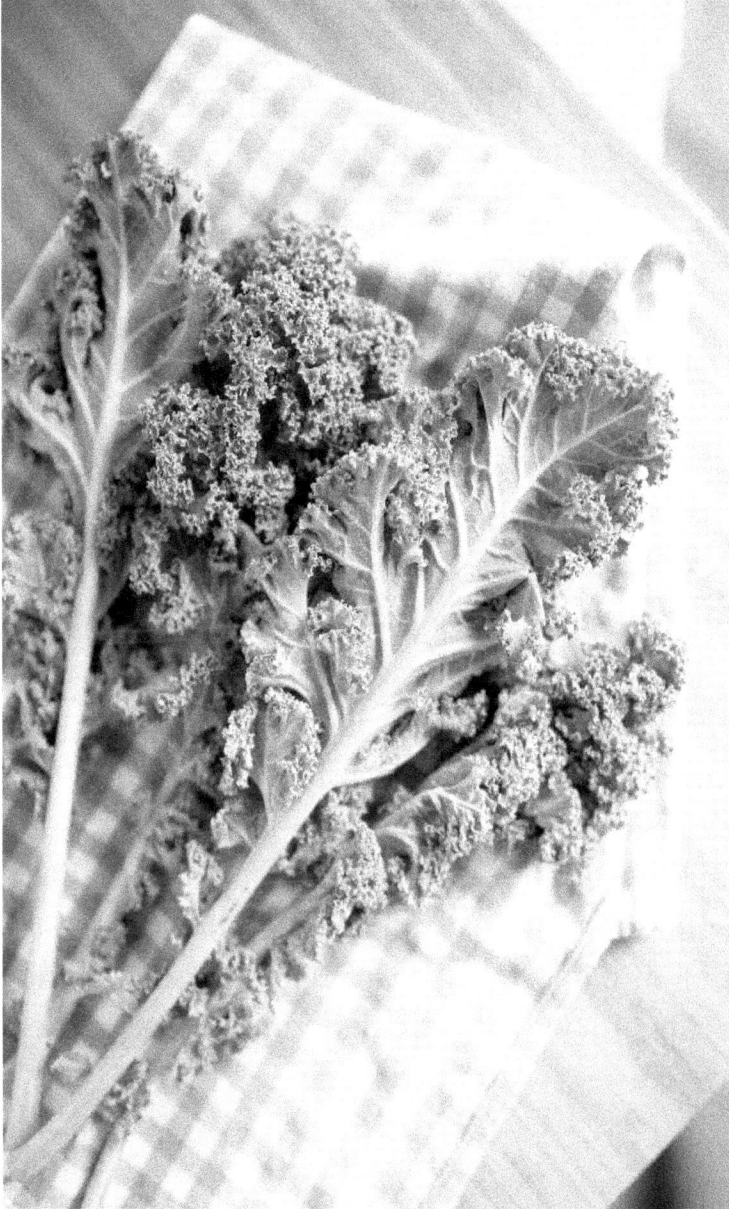

Chapter 4

Nutritional Strategies

Foods that promote eye health

Proper nutrition plays a crucial role in maintaining good eye health and preventing cataracts. There are certain foods that are known to promote eye health and reduce the risk of developing cataracts. Including these foods in your diet can help protect your vision and maintain clear eyesight for years to come.

One of the most important nutrients for eye health is lutein and zeaxanthin, which are found in high concentrations in leafy green vegetables such as spinach, kale, and collard greens. These antioxidants help protect the eyes from harmful UV rays and reduce the risk of cataracts. Adding these vegetables to your diet can provide a natural defense against cataract formation.

Another important nutrient for eye health is vitamin C, which is found in citrus fruits, strawberries, and bell peppers. Vitamin C helps strengthen the eye's blood vessels and reduce the risk of cataracts. Including these foods in your diet can help maintain healthy eyes and prevent vision problems as you age.

Omega-3 fatty acids are also essential for eye health and can be found in fatty fish such as salmon, mackerel, and sardines. These healthy fats help reduce inflammation in the eyes and protect against cataract formation. Adding fish to your diet a few times a week can provide a significant boost to your eye health and overall well-being.

In addition to including these foods in your diet, it is also important to stay hydrated and drink plenty of water throughout the day. Proper hydration helps maintain the moisture levels in the eyes and prevents dryness, which can contribute to cataract formation. By making small changes to your diet and lifestyle, you can promote good eye health and reduce the risk of developing cataracts in the future.

Vitamins and supplements for cataract prevention

Vitamins and supplements can play a crucial role in preventing cataracts, which are a common age-related eye condition that can lead to vision loss if left untreated.

By incorporating certain nutrients into your diet or taking supplements, you can help reduce your risk of developing cataracts and maintain clear vision for longer.

One of the most important vitamins for cataract prevention is vitamin C. This powerful antioxidant helps protect the eyes from oxidative stress and damage caused by free radicals. Foods rich in vitamin C include citrus fruits, red bell peppers, and strawberries.

Alternatively, you can take a vitamin C supplement to ensure you are getting an adequate amount of this essential nutrient.

Vitamin E is another key nutrient for preventing cataracts. Like vitamin C, vitamin E is an antioxidant that helps protect the eyes from damage. Nuts, seeds, and leafy green vegetables are all excellent sources of vitamin E. Taking a vitamin E supplement can also be beneficial in reducing your risk of developing cataracts.

In addition to vitamins C and E, lutein and zeaxanthin are two important nutrients for cataract prevention. These carotenoids are found in high concentrations in the eyes and help filter out harmful blue light. Foods such as spinach, kale, and eggs are rich sources of lutein and zeaxanthin. If you have difficulty getting enough of these nutrients from your diet, consider taking a supplement to support your eye health.

Overall, maintaining a balanced diet rich in vitamins and nutrients is essential for cataract prevention. By incorporating foods high in vitamin C, vitamin E, lutein, and zeaxanthin into your daily meals, you can help protect your eyes from cataracts and maintain clear vision as you age.

Remember to consult with your eye care professional before starting any new supplement regimen to ensure it is safe and appropriate for your individual needs.

Hydration and its impact on eye health

Proper hydration plays a crucial role in maintaining overall health, including the health of your eyes. Dehydration can lead to a number of health issues, including dry eyes, which can contribute to the development of cataracts. When your body is dehydrated, it can affect the production of tears, causing dryness and irritation in the eyes. Staying adequately hydrated by drinking plenty of water throughout the day can help prevent dry eyes and protect the health of your eyes.

In addition to preventing dry eyes, staying properly hydrated can also help reduce the risk of developing cataracts. Cataracts are a common age-related eye condition that causes cloudy vision and can eventually lead to blindness if left untreated.

By keeping your body well-hydrated, you can help maintain the health of your eyes and reduce the risk of developing cataracts as you age. Drinking water regularly can also help flush out toxins from your body, which can have a positive impact on your eye health.

It's important to note that not all fluids are created equal when it comes to hydration and eye health. While sugary drinks and caffeinated beverages can contribute to dehydration, water is the best choice for maintaining proper hydration levels. Aim to drink at least eight glasses of water a day to keep your body and eyes properly hydrated. If you struggle to drink enough water throughout the day, try carrying a reusable water bottle with you and setting reminders to take sips regularly.

In addition to drinking water, eating a diet rich in hydrating foods can also help support eye health and prevent cataracts. Foods like cucumbers, watermelon, and oranges are high in water content and can help keep your body hydrated. Incorporating these hydrating foods into your diet can provide additional support for your eye health and overall well-being.

By focusing on hydration through both water intake and hydrating foods, you can help protect your eyes from the development of cataracts and other age-related eye conditions.

In conclusion, maintaining proper hydration is essential for supporting eye health and preventing the development of cataracts. By drinking plenty of water, eating hydrating foods, and avoiding dehydrating beverages, you can help keep your eyes healthy and reduce the risk of developing cataracts as you age. Making hydration a priority in your daily routine is a simple yet effective way to protect your vision and maintain clear, healthy eyes for years to come.

How To Prevent Cataracts

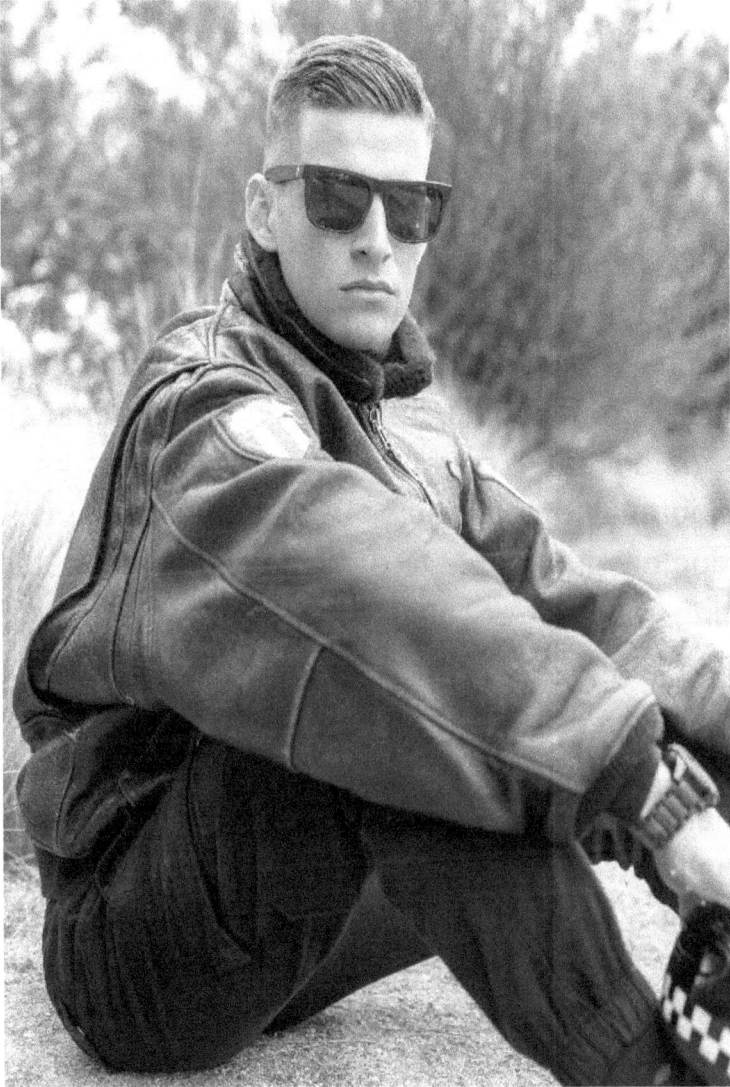

Chapter 5

Vision Care Practices

Regular eye exams

Regular eye exams are crucial in the prevention of cataracts. By scheduling routine appointments with an eye care professional, you can catch any changes in your vision early on and take steps to prevent the development of cataracts. During these exams, your eye doctor will be able to detect any signs of cataracts forming and offer advice on how to slow their progression.

One of the key benefits of regular eye exams is the early detection of cataracts. By catching cataracts in their early stages, you have a better chance of preventing them from worsening and impacting your vision. Your eye doctor will be able to monitor the progression of cataracts and recommend treatment options to help preserve your vision for as long as possible.

In addition to detecting cataracts, regular eye exams also allow your eye care professional to assess your overall eye health. They can identify any other eye conditions or diseases that may be present, such as macular degeneration or glaucoma. By addressing these issues early on, you can prevent further damage to your eyes and maintain clear vision for years to come.

Furthermore, regular eye exams are an important part of maintaining your overall health and well-being. Many systemic health conditions, such as diabetes and high blood pressure, can impact your eye health and increase your risk of developing cataracts. By monitoring your eye health through regular exams, you can catch these conditions early and take steps to manage them effectively.

In conclusion, regular eye exams play a vital role in the prevention of cataracts and maintaining clear vision. By scheduling routine appointments with your doctor, you can detect cataracts early, assess your overall eye health, and address any underlying health conditions that may impact your vision. Take control of your eye health today by making regular eye exams a priority in your preventive care routine.

Proper eyewear for eye protection

Proper eyewear for eye protection is essential for preventing cataracts. Cataracts are a common eye condition that can lead to blurred vision and even blindness if left untreated. One of the most effective ways to prevent cataracts is by wearing the right kind of eyewear to protect your eyes from harmful UV rays and other environmental factors.

When it comes to choosing the right eyewear for eye protection, it's important to opt for sunglasses that offer 100% UV protection. UV rays from the sun can damage the proteins in the lens of your eye, leading to the formation of cataracts over time. By wearing sunglasses with UV protection, you can help prevent this damage and reduce your risk of developing cataracts.

In addition to UV protection, it's also important to choose sunglasses that provide adequate coverage for your eyes. Wrap-around sunglasses are a good option as they provide protection from all angles, including the sides. This can help shield your eyes from the sun's rays and reduce your risk of developing cataracts.

For those who spend a lot of time outdoors, polarized sunglasses can be particularly beneficial. Polarized lenses reduce glare and improve contrast, making it easier to see in bright sunlight. This can help reduce eye strain and further protect your eyes from the harmful effects of UV rays.

Overall, wearing proper eyewear for eye protection is a simple yet effective way to prevent cataracts and maintain clear vision. By choosing sunglasses with 100% UV protection, adequate coverage, and polarization, you can help protect your eyes and reduce your risk of developing this common eye condition. Investing in quality eyewear is an investment in your eye health and can help you enjoy clear vision for years to come.

Resting and relaxing your eyes

Resting and relaxing your eyes is an important aspect of preventing cataracts. Many people don't realize the strain that constant use of digital devices and screens can have on their eyes. Taking regular breaks from staring at screens and focusing on distant objects can help reduce this strain and prevent cataracts from developing.

One simple way to rest and relax your eyes is to practice the 20-20-20 rule. This rule suggests that every 20 minutes, you should take a 20-second break and look at something 20 feet away. This allows your eyes to relax and refocus, reducing the strain that can lead to cataracts.

In addition to taking regular breaks, it's important to make sure you are getting enough sleep. Lack of sleep can contribute to eye strain and increase your risk of developing cataracts. Aim for at least 7-8 hours of quality sleep each night to give your eyes the rest they need to stay healthy.

Another way to rest and relax your eyes is to practice eye exercises. These exercises can help strengthen the muscles in your eyes and improve your overall eye health. Simple exercises like blinking, rolling your eyes, and focusing on different objects can help reduce eye strain and prevent cataracts from forming.

By incorporating these simple strategies into your daily routine, you can help prevent cataracts and maintain clear vision for years to come. Remember to take breaks, get plenty of sleep, and practice eye exercises regularly to keep your eyes healthy and cataract-free.

How To Prevent Cataracts

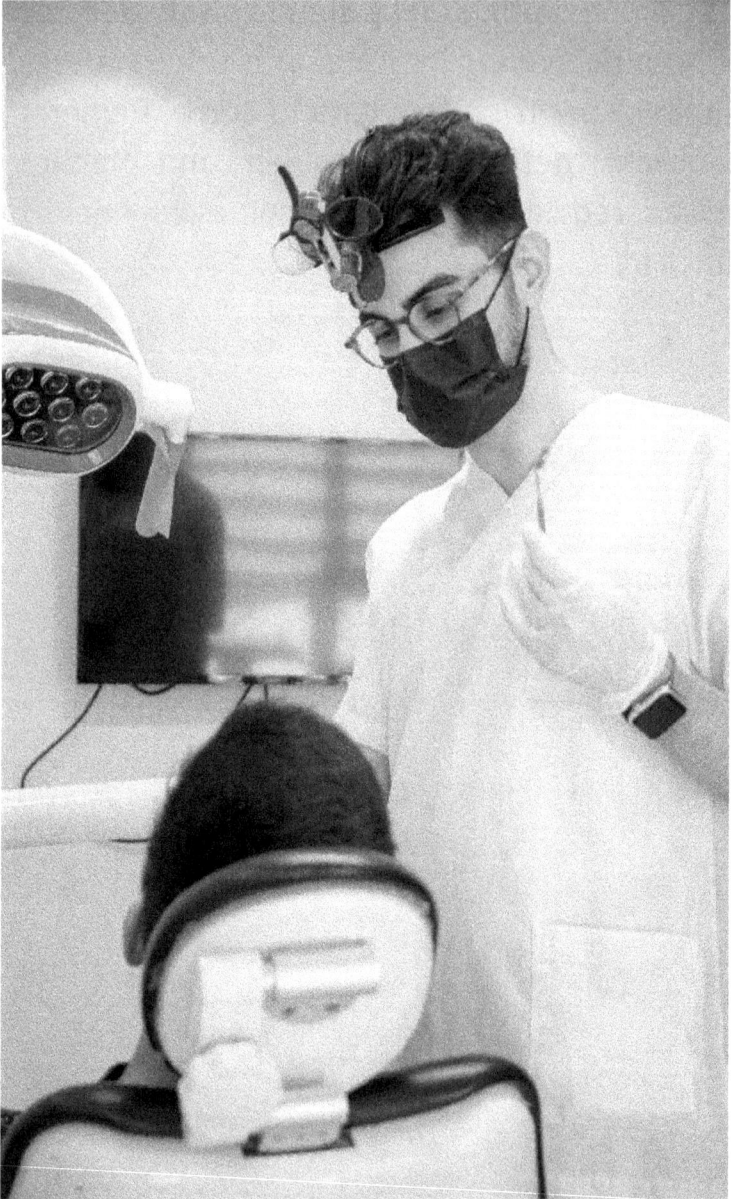

Chapter 6

Environmental Factors to Consider

Avoiding smoking and secondhand smoke

Smoking and exposure to secondhand smoke have been linked to an increased risk of developing cataracts. Cataracts are a common vision problem that can lead to cloudy or blurry vision, making it difficult to see clearly. By avoiding smoking and limiting your exposure to secondhand smoke, you can help reduce your risk of developing cataracts and maintain clear vision for longer.

Smoking is a well-known risk factor for cataracts, as the chemicals in cigarettes can cause damage to the lens of the eye over time. This damage can lead to the development of cataracts, which can significantly impact your vision and quality of life. By quitting smoking or never starting in the first place, you can greatly reduce your risk of developing cataracts and other eye problems.

In addition to avoiding smoking, it is also important to limit your exposure to secondhand smoke. Secondhand smoke contains many of the same harmful chemicals as firsthand smoke, and can still put you at risk for developing cataracts and other eye conditions.

By avoiding places where smoking is allowed and asking those around you not to smoke indoors or in enclosed spaces, you can help protect your eyes and reduce your risk of cataracts.

If you are concerned about cataracts and want to take steps to prevent them, avoiding smoking and secondhand smoke is an important first step. By making healthy lifestyle choices and avoiding harmful substances like tobacco smoke, you can reduce your risk of developing cataracts and maintain clear vision for years to come.

Remember, your eye health is important, and taking steps to protect your eyes now can help prevent vision problems later in life.

Managing diabetes and other health conditions

Managing diabetes and other health conditions is crucial for preventing the development of cataracts. Diabetes is a known risk factor for cataracts, as high blood sugar levels can cause damage to the lens of the eye. It is important for individuals with diabetes to closely monitor their blood sugar levels and follow a healthy diet and exercise routine to help prevent cataracts from forming.

In addition to diabetes, other health conditions such as high blood pressure and obesity can also increase the risk of developing cataracts. Managing these conditions through proper medical treatment and lifestyle changes can help reduce the risk of cataracts.

It is important for individuals to work closely with their healthcare providers to develop a comprehensive treatment plan that addresses all of their health concerns.

Regular eye exams are essential for individuals with diabetes and other health conditions, as they can help identify early signs of cataracts and other eye problems.

By detecting cataracts early, treatment options can be explored to help preserve vision and prevent further damage to the eyes. Individuals should make it a priority to schedule annual eye exams with an eye care professional to monitor their eye health and address any concerns.

In addition to managing health conditions, individuals can also take steps to protect their eyes from harmful ultraviolet (UV) rays and other environmental factors that can contribute to cataract development. Wearing sunglasses that block 100% of UV rays and hats with brims can help shield the eyes from the sun's harmful rays.

Additionally, individuals should avoid smoking and limit alcohol consumption, as these habits can also increase the risk of cataracts.

By taking proactive steps to manage diabetes and other health conditions, individuals can reduce their risk of developing cataracts and maintain clear vision for years to come.

It is important for individuals to prioritize their eye health and work closely with healthcare providers to develop a comprehensive plan for managing their overall health and preventing cataracts. With proper care and attention, individuals can protect their vision and enjoy a lifetime of clear sight.

Limiting exposure to toxins and pollutants

Cataracts are a common eye condition that can lead to blurry vision and, in severe cases, blindness. While genetics play a role in the development of cataracts, exposure to toxins and pollutants can also increase your risk. In this subchapter, we will discuss strategies for limiting your exposure to these harmful substances to help prevent cataracts and protect your vision.

How To Prevent Cataracts

One of the most important steps you can take to limit your exposure to toxins and pollutants is to be mindful of the products you use in your home. Many household cleaners, pesticides, and personal care products contain harmful chemicals that can contribute to cataract formation. Choosing natural, eco-friendly alternatives can help reduce your risk of exposure and protect your eye health.

In addition to being mindful of the products you use, it is also important to pay attention to the air quality in your environment. Air pollution, both indoors and outdoors, can contain toxins and pollutants that can harm your eyes. Using air purifiers in your home, avoiding smoking and secondhand smoke, and limiting your time spent in areas with poor air quality can all help reduce your risk of cataracts.

Another important factor to consider when trying to limit your exposure to toxins and pollutants is your diet. Eating a healthy, balanced diet rich in antioxidants can help protect your eyes from damage caused by free radicals, which are harmful substances that can contribute to cataract formation. Foods like leafy greens, berries, and nuts are all good sources of antioxidants that can help keep your eyes healthy.

Finally, it is important to stay informed about potential sources of toxins and pollutants in your environment. Keeping up to date on local air quality reports, avoiding areas with high levels of pollution, and staying informed about potential toxins in your water supply can all help you make informed decisions to protect your eye health. By taking these steps to limit your exposure to harmful substances, you can help prevent cataracts and maintain clear vision for years to come.

How To Prevent Cataracts

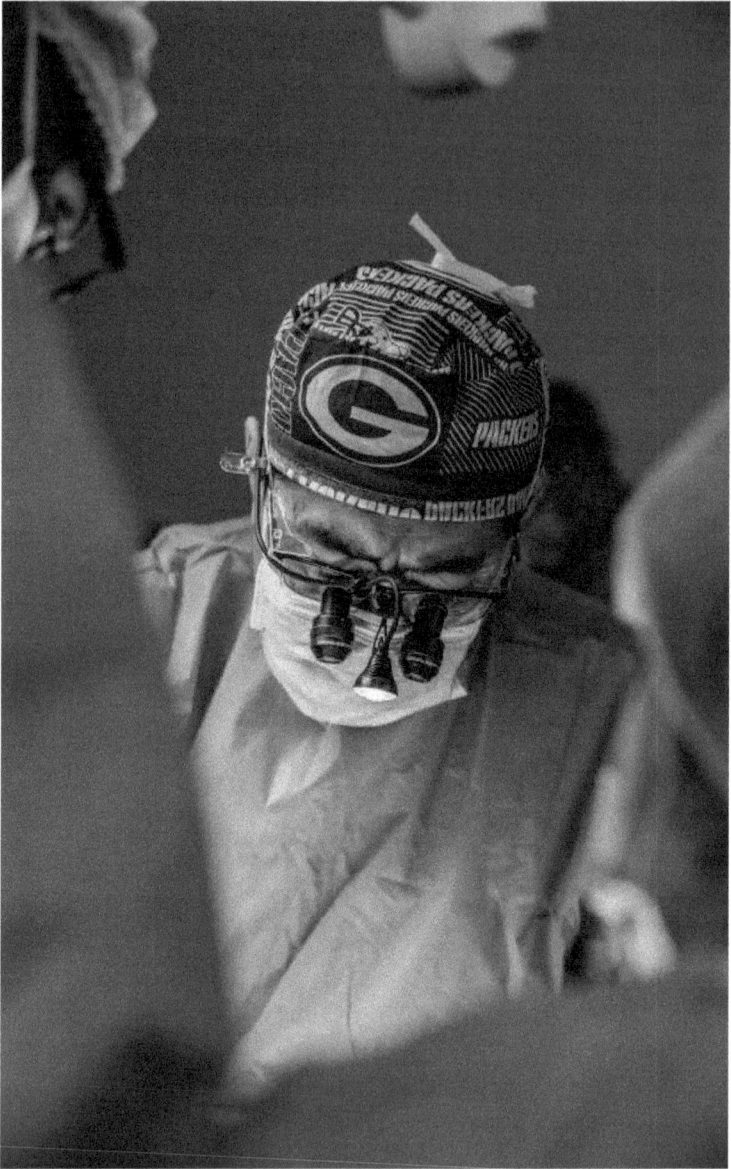

Chapter 7

Surgical Options for Cataracts

Understanding cataract surgery

Cataract surgery is a common procedure performed to remove a cloudy lens in the eye that is causing vision problems. Understanding the process of cataract surgery can help alleviate any fears or concerns you may have about the procedure. In this subchapter, we will delve into the details of cataract surgery and provide you with the information you need to make an informed decision about your eye health.

During cataract surgery, the cloudy lens in your eye is removed and replaced with a clear artificial lens. This procedure is typically done on an outpatient basis, meaning you can go home the same day. The surgery itself is relatively quick, usually taking less than an hour to complete. Most patients report minimal discomfort during the procedure, and the recovery time is usually short.

Before undergoing cataract surgery, your eye doctor will perform a thorough eye exam to determine the severity of your cataracts and assess your overall eye health. You will also have the opportunity to discuss any concerns or questions you may have about the procedure. It is important to follow your doctor's pre-operative instructions to ensure the best possible outcome for your surgery.

After cataract surgery, you may experience some mild discomfort and blurry vision for a few days. Your doctor will provide you with instructions on how to care for your eyes post-surgery, including using prescription eye drops and avoiding strenuous activities. Most patients notice an improvement in their vision within a few days of the surgery and are able to resume normal activities shortly thereafter.

In conclusion, cataract surgery is a safe and effective procedure that can improve your vision and quality of life. By understanding the process of cataract surgery and being informed about what to expect before, during, and after the procedure, you can approach the surgery with confidence and peace of mind.

If you have concerns about cataracts or are considering cataract surgery, be sure to consult with your eye doctor to discuss your options and develop a treatment plan that is right for you.

Preparing for surgery

Preparing for surgery is an important step in ensuring a successful outcome for cataract treatment. Before undergoing cataract surgery, it is essential to follow some key steps to ensure that you are fully prepared for the procedure.

The first step is to schedule a consultation with your ophthalmologist to discuss the details of the surgery and address any concerns or questions you may have. During this consultation, your doctor will also perform a thorough eye exam to determine the severity of your cataracts and assess your overall eye health.

Following your consultation, your doctor may provide you with specific instructions to follow in the days leading up to your surgery. These instructions may include guidelines on when to stop eating or drinking before the procedure, as well as any medications you should avoid taking in the days leading up to surgery. It is important to follow these instructions closely to ensure that you are in the best possible physical condition for the surgery.

In addition to following your doctor's instructions, it is also important to make any necessary arrangements for the day of the surgery. This may include arranging for transportation to and from the surgical facility, as well as making arrangements for someone to accompany you to the appointment.

You may also need to make arrangements for any post-operative care that may be necessary, such as ensuring that you have someone available to assist you with daily tasks while you recover.

Finally, it is important to maintain a positive attitude and mindset leading up to your surgery. While cataract surgery is a routine procedure with a high success rate, it is normal to feel anxious or nervous about undergoing surgery. Remember that your ophthalmologist is experienced and skilled in performing cataract surgery and will take all necessary precautions to ensure a safe and successful procedure. By following these steps and maintaining a positive attitude, you can ensure that you are fully prepared for cataract surgery and set yourself up for a successful outcome and clear vision.

Recovery and post-operative care

Recovery and post-operative care are crucial aspects of the cataract surgery process. Following the procedure, it is important to take the necessary steps to ensure a smooth and successful recovery. Your eye doctor will provide you with specific instructions on how to care for your eyes in the days and weeks following surgery. It is important to follow these instructions closely to promote healing and minimize the risk of complications.

One of the key aspects of post-operative care is the use of prescribed eye drops. These drops help to prevent infection, reduce inflammation, and promote healing. It is important to use the drops as directed by your doctor, even if your eyes feel fine. Skipping doses or stopping treatment prematurely can increase the risk of complications and delay healing. Make sure to wash your hands thoroughly before administering the drops to prevent introducing bacteria into the eye.

During the recovery period, it is important to avoid activities that could put your eyes at risk of injury or infection. This includes avoiding rubbing or touching your eyes, as well as staying away from dusty or dirty environments.

It is also important to avoid swimming or using hot tubs during the first few weeks after surgery, as water can introduce bacteria into the eyes. Your doctor may also recommend wearing a protective shield over your eye at night to prevent accidental rubbing or scratching.

It is normal to experience some discomfort, redness, or sensitivity to light in the days following cataract surgery. These symptoms should improve as your eyes heal, but it is important to contact your doctor if you experience severe pain, sudden vision changes, or any other concerning symptoms. Your doctor will schedule follow-up appointments to monitor your progress and ensure that your eyes are healing properly. Be sure to attend these appointments and follow any additional instructions provided by your doctor.

In most cases, patients are able to resume their normal activities within a few days to a week after cataract surgery. However, it is important to listen to your body and give yourself time to rest and recover. Avoid strenuous activities, heavy lifting, or bending over for extended periods of time in the days following surgery. By following your doctor's instructions and taking good care of your eyes during the recovery period, you can help ensure a successful outcome and enjoy clear vision for years to come.

How To Prevent Cataracts

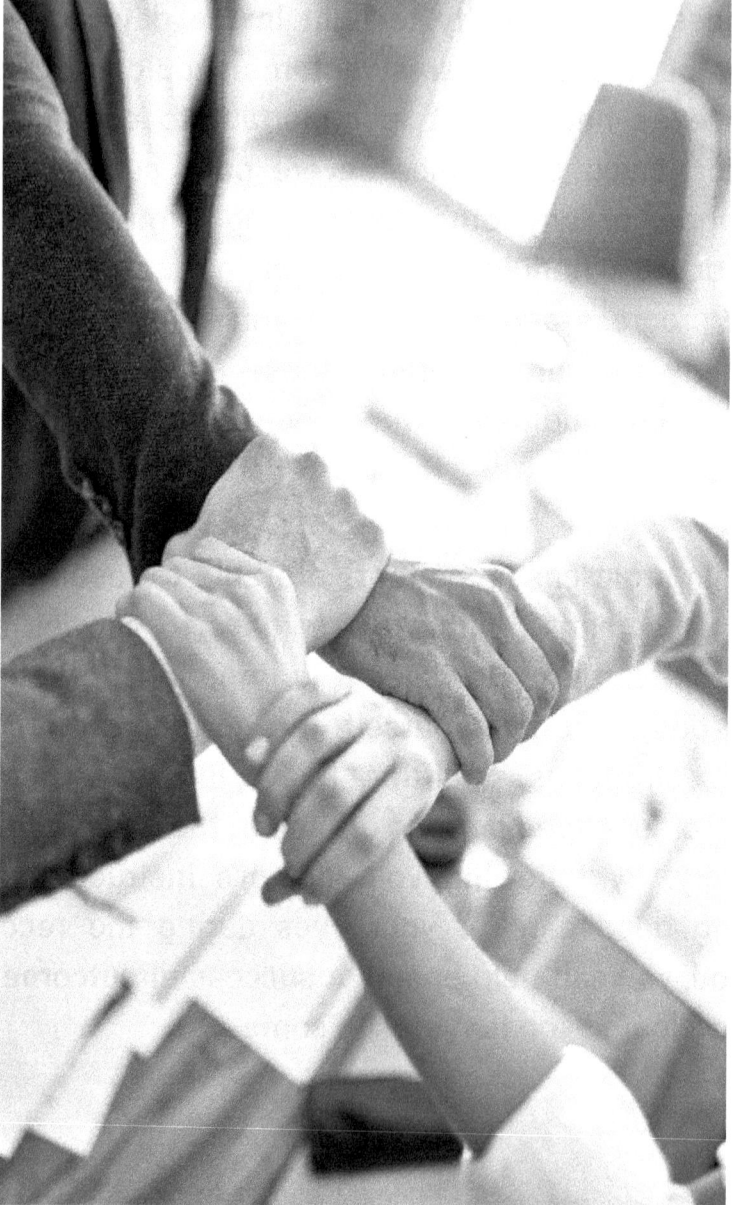

Strategies for Clear Vision

Chapter 8

Support and Resources

Joining support groups for cataract patients

Support groups for cataract patients can be incredibly beneficial for those who are concerned about cataracts and looking for ways to prevent them. By joining a support group, individuals can connect with others who are going through similar experiences and share advice, tips, and resources for maintaining clear vision. These groups often provide a sense of community and understanding that can help individuals feel less alone in their journey to prevent cataracts.

One of the key benefits of joining a support group for cataract patients is the opportunity to learn from others who have successfully prevented or managed their cataracts. Members of these groups can share their personal stories, treatment options, and lifestyle changes that have helped them maintain clear vision.

By listening to these experiences, individuals can gain valuable insights and strategies for preventing cataracts in their own lives.

Support groups for cataract patients also provide a platform for individuals to ask questions and seek advice from others who have firsthand experience with the condition. Whether it's about dietary changes, eye exercises, or alternative therapies, members of these groups can offer guidance and support to help individuals make informed decisions about their eye health. This exchange of information can be invaluable in empowering individuals to take proactive steps towards preventing cataracts.

In addition to sharing knowledge and experiences, support groups for cataract patients can also serve as a source of emotional support and encouragement. Dealing with the fear and uncertainty of developing cataracts can be overwhelming, but knowing that there are others who understand and empathize with your struggles can provide a sense of comfort and reassurance. By connecting with a community of like-minded individuals, individuals can feel supported and motivated to take charge of their eye health and prevent cataracts.

Overall, joining a support group for cataract patients can be a valuable resource for individuals who are concerned about cataracts and interested in preventing them. These groups offer a sense of community, knowledge sharing, emotional support, and encouragement that can help individuals navigate their journey towards clear vision.

By connecting with others who share similar goals and experiences, individuals can gain the tools and motivation they need to take proactive steps towards preventing cataracts and maintaining healthy eyesight for years to come.

Finding financial assistance for cataract treatment

Cataracts are a common eye condition that affects millions of people worldwide. While cataract surgery is the most effective treatment for cataracts, it can be costly and not always covered by insurance. For those who are concerned about the financial burden of cataract treatment, there are options available to help offset the costs.

One option for financial assistance for cataract treatment is to check with your insurance provider to see what coverage is available for cataract surgery. Some insurance plans may cover all or part of the cost of cataract surgery, depending on the specific plan and the severity of the cataracts.

It is important to review your insurance policy and speak with your provider to understand what is covered and what out-of-pocket expenses you may incur.

If your insurance does not cover cataract surgery or if you do not have insurance, there are other resources available to help with the cost of treatment. Some hospitals and clinics offer financial assistance programs for patients who cannot afford cataract surgery.

These programs may be based on income eligibility or other criteria, so it is important to inquire with the hospital or clinic where you plan to have the surgery to see if you qualify for financial assistance.

Another option for financial assistance for cataract treatment is to explore government programs that provide assistance for medical expenses. Programs such as Medicaid or Medicare may cover cataract surgery for eligible individuals.

Additionally, there are nonprofit organizations that provide financial assistance for eye care and cataract surgery for those in need. These organizations may have specific eligibility requirements, so it is important to research and reach out to them for more information.

In conclusion, finding financial assistance for cataract treatment is possible for those who are concerned about the costs associated with cataract surgery. By exploring options such as insurance coverage, hospital financial assistance programs, government programs, and nonprofit organizations, individuals can find the resources they need to help offset the costs of cataract treatment.

It is important to research and inquire about these options to ensure that you receive the financial assistance you need for clear vision and improved eye health.

Additional resources for cataract prevention

Cataracts are a common eye condition that can significantly impact your vision as you age. While there is no guaranteed way to prevent cataracts from developing, there are several strategies you can incorporate into your daily routine to reduce your risk. In addition to maintaining a healthy diet and wearing sunglasses to protect your eyes from UV rays, there are several additional resources available to help you prevent cataracts.

One valuable resource for cataract prevention is regular eye exams. By scheduling eye exams with an optometrist or ophthalmologist on a yearly basis, you can catch any signs of cataracts early on and receive timely treatment. Early detection is key in managing cataracts and preventing them from worsening over time. Additionally, eye exams can help identify other eye conditions that may increase your risk of developing cataracts.

Another helpful resource for cataract prevention is staying informed about the latest research and developments in eye health. By staying up-to-date on current studies and recommendations from reputable sources such as the American Academy of Ophthalmology or the National Eye Institute, you can make informed decisions about your eye care and take proactive steps to prevent cataracts. Many organizations offer educational materials and resources on cataract prevention that can help you better understand the condition and how to reduce your risk.

In addition to regular eye exams and staying informed, maintaining a healthy lifestyle can also play a significant role in cataract prevention. Eating a diet rich in antioxidants, vitamins, and minerals can help protect your eyes from cataracts and other age-related eye conditions. Exercise, quitting smoking, and managing underlying health conditions such as diabetes can also help reduce your risk of developing cataracts. By taking a holistic approach to your health and wellness, you can support your eye health and potentially prevent cataracts from developing.

Overall, there are many resources available to help you prevent cataracts and preserve your vision as you age. By incorporating regular eye exams, staying informed about eye health, and maintaining a healthy lifestyle, you can take proactive steps to reduce your risk of developing cataracts. Remember that prevention is key when it comes to cataracts, and by taking control of your eye health, you can enjoy clear vision for years to come.

How To Prevent Cataracts

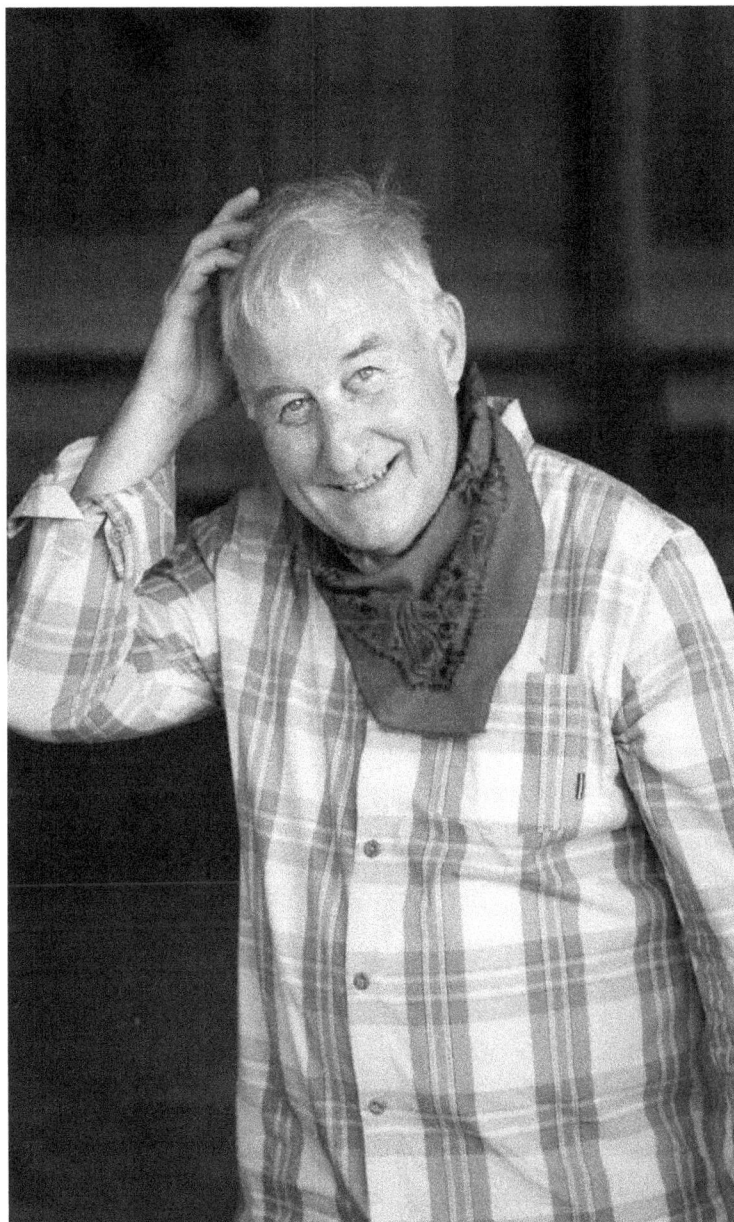

Chapter 9

Conclusion

Recap of key strategies for preventing cataracts

Cataracts are a common eye condition that can greatly impact one's vision if left untreated. In order to prevent cataracts from developing, there are several key strategies that individuals can incorporate into their daily routine. Understanding these strategies and implementing them consistently can help to reduce the risk of cataracts and maintain clear vision for years to come.

One of the most important strategies for preventing cataracts is to protect your eyes from harmful UV rays. This can be done by wearing sunglasses that block out 100% of UVA and UVB rays whenever you are outdoors, especially during peak sun hours. UV exposure has been linked to the development of cataracts, so it is essential to take this precaution to safeguard your eye health.

Another key strategy for preventing cataracts is to eat a healthy diet rich in antioxidants and vitamins. Foods such as leafy greens, citrus fruits, and berries are high in antioxidants that can help to protect the eyes from oxidative stress and damage. Including these foods in your daily meals can provide essential nutrients that support eye health and reduce the risk of cataracts.

Maintaining a healthy lifestyle that includes regular exercise and avoiding smoking can also play a significant role in preventing cataracts. Exercise helps to improve circulation and reduce inflammation, which can benefit overall eye health. Smoking, on the other hand, has been linked to an increased risk of cataracts, so quitting this habit can greatly reduce your chances of developing the condition.

Regular eye exams are another important strategy for preventing cataracts. By seeing an eye care professional on a routine basis, any early signs of cataracts can be detected and addressed before they progress. Early intervention is key in managing cataracts and preserving clear vision, so it is essential to prioritize regular eye check-ups as part of your preventive care routine.

In conclusion, by incorporating these key strategies into your daily routine, you can take proactive steps to prevent cataracts and maintain clear vision for years to come. From protecting your eyes from UV rays to eating a healthy diet and staying active, there are many ways to reduce your risk of developing cataracts. By prioritizing your eye health and following these preventive measures, you can take control of your vision and enjoy clear, healthy eyes for a lifetime.

Encouragement for maintaining healthy vision

Maintaining healthy vision is crucial for overall well-being, especially for those who are concerned about cataracts. Cataracts are a common eye condition that can lead to blurry vision and difficulty seeing clearly. However, there are steps you can take to prevent cataracts and maintain healthy vision for years to come. By following a few simple guidelines, you can reduce your risk of developing cataracts and enjoy clear vision for a lifetime.

One of the most important things you can do to maintain healthy vision and prevent cataracts is to eat a balanced diet rich in fruits and vegetables. Foods that are high in antioxidants, such as leafy greens, citrus fruits, and berries, can help protect your eyes from damage caused by free radicals. Additionally, incorporating foods high in vitamins C and E, zinc, and omega-3 fatty acids into your diet can also help maintain healthy vision and reduce your risk of developing cataracts.

Another key factor in maintaining healthy vision is to protect your eyes from harmful UV rays. Prolonged exposure to the sun's ultraviolet rays can increase your risk of developing cataracts, so it's important to wear sunglasses that block 100% of UVA and UVB rays whenever you're outside. Additionally, wearing a wide-brimmed hat can provide added protection for your eyes and help reduce your risk of developing cataracts.

Regular eye exams are also essential for maintaining healthy vision and preventing cataracts. By having your eyes checked regularly by an eye care professional, you can catch any potential issues early and take steps to address them before they progress.

Your eye doctor can also provide guidance on lifestyle changes you can make to reduce your risk of developing cataracts and other eye conditions.

In addition to these lifestyle changes, it's important to avoid smoking and limit alcohol consumption, as both can increase your risk of developing cataracts. By making these simple changes to your daily routine and following the advice of your eye care professional, you can maintain healthy vision and reduce your risk of developing cataracts as you age.

Remember, your eyes are precious, so take steps to protect them and enjoy clear vision for years to come.

Looking towards a future free from cataracts

As we look towards a future free from cataracts, it is important to understand the risk factors and preventative measures that can help us maintain clear vision as we age. Cataracts are a common age-related eye condition that can cause blurred vision, sensitivity to light, and difficulty seeing at night.

By taking proactive steps to protect our eye health, we can reduce our risk of developing cataracts and enjoy clear vision for years to come.

One of the most important strategies for preventing cataracts is to protect our eyes from harmful UV rays. Prolonged exposure to sunlight can increase the risk of developing cataracts, so it is essential to wear sunglasses that block out 100% of UVA and UVB rays whenever we are outdoors.

Additionally, wearing a wide-brimmed hat can provide added protection for our eyes and help to reduce the risk of cataract formation.

In addition to protecting our eyes from UV rays, maintaining a healthy diet and lifestyle can also play a significant role in preventing cataracts. Eating a diet rich in antioxidants, such as fruits and vegetables, can help to protect our eyes from oxidative damage and reduce the risk of cataracts.

Regular exercise, not smoking, and maintaining a healthy weight are also important factors in preventing cataracts and maintaining overall eye health.

Regular eye exams are another crucial component of preventing cataracts and catching any potential issues early on. By scheduling regular appointments with an eye care professional, we can monitor our eye health and address any concerns before they develop into more serious problems. Early detection and treatment are key in preventing cataracts and preserving our vision for the future.

How To Prevent Cataracts

By taking proactive steps to protect our eyes, maintain a healthy lifestyle, and schedule regular eye exams, we can work towards a future free from cataracts. With the right strategies and preventative measures in place, we can reduce our risk of developing cataracts and enjoy clear vision well into our golden years. Let us take control of our eye health today and look towards a future with clear, cataract-free vision.

Author Notes & Acknowledgments

First and foremost, I would like to express my deepest gratitude to the people who inspired and supported me throughout the journey of writing this book. This project would not have been possible without their unwavering belief in me and their invaluable contributions.

To my wife, thank you for your constant encouragement and understanding. Your love and support have been my anchor during the challenging times of researching and writing this book. Your belief in my ability to make a difference in people's lives has been my driving force.

I would also like to disclose that this book contains some renewed artificial intelligence-generated content. I really appreciate very recent technological innovation by outstanding scientists and of course our reader's understanding.

Lastly, I want to express my deepest gratitude to the readers of this book. I sincerely hope the strategies and methods outlined within these pages will provide you with the knowledge and tools needed to truly make your life much better. Your commitment to seeking any good solutions and willingness to explore multiple methods is commendable.

Author Bio

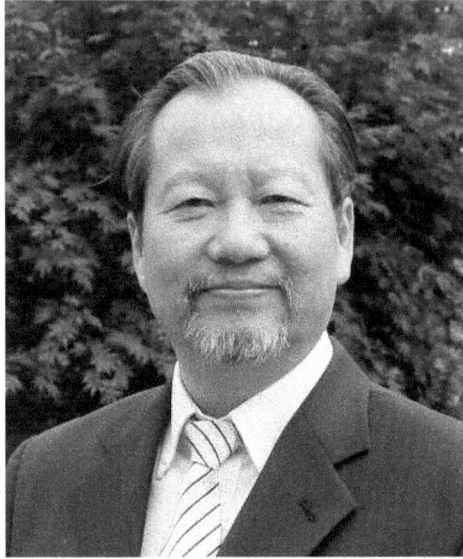

Johnson Wu earned his MD in 1982. With over 40 years of clinical experience, he has worked in hospitals in Zhejiang and Shanghai, China, as well as the Royal Marsden Hospital (part of Imperial College) in London, UK.

Upon the recommendation of Sir Aaron Klug, the president of The Royal Society and a Nobel Prize winner in Chemistry, Dr. Wu was honorably awarded a British Royal Society Fellowship. He has published medical books and articles in seven countries and currently practices medicine in Canada.

www.ingramcontent.com/pod-product-compliance
Lightning Source LLC
Chambersburg PA
CBHW060256030426
42335CB00014B/1723